DIY Healing Salve:
20 Recipes Of Healing Salves For All-Purpose Use

Disclamer: All photos used in this book, including the cover photo were made available under a Attribution-NonCommercial-ShareAlike 2.0 Generic and sourced from Flickr

Table of content

Introduction 4
Chapter 1 – Tips to Make Herbal Salves 6
Chapter 2 – 20 Herbal Salve Recipes for Various Uses 14
Recipe 01: Standard Salve 14
Recipe 02: All-purpose Healing Salve 15
Recipe 03: Basic Recipe for Salve 16
Recipe 04: First Aid Salve 17
Recipe 05: Diaper Rash Salve 17
Recipe 06: Burn Salve 18
Recipe 07: Cuticle Balm 19
Recipe 08: Herbal Infused Balm 20
Recipe 09: Foot Salve 20
Recipe 10: Charcoal Black Salve 21
Recipe 11: Perfect Salve for Burn 22
Recipe 12: Plantain Salve 22
Recipe 13: Dandelion Salve 23
Recipe 14: Sore Muscles Salve 23
Recipe 15: Pepper Salve for Joint and Arthritis 25
Recipe 16: Chest Rub 25
Recipe 17: Hemorrhoid Salve 26
Recipe 18: Salve for Gardener 26
Recipe 19: Lip Salve 27

Recipe 20: Super-Strength Salve for Pain 27

Conclusion 29

Introduction

Herbal salves enable you to get the benefit of healing powers of various herbs. It is useful for the treatment of cuts, infections, bruises and other similar problems. You should have these salves in your cabinet because of their benefits. Use of herbal salve can help you to get rid of various health conditions, such as:

Infection

Herbal salves have healing abilities, and you can use it to treat infections, including boils. These are helpful to bring infection out of your boil and relieve discomfort and speed healing process of the boil. Some salves have antibacterial and antifungal properties. These are good to prevent infection of cuts and minor scrapes.

Soothing Salves

You can use salves to soothe irritated or chap skin. Salves and lip balms are good to treat rashes. These are good for the whole family to get rid of various skin irritations. Fortunately, you can make these salves at home without any problem.

Salves are helpful for the treatment of arthritis pain, splinters, and insect bites. You can even use them to treat allergies and cold. You should carry a tube of herbal salve with you to address minor illnesses. Keep it in mind that these herbs are precious for everyone to deal with various conditions. Make these salves at home with natural ingredients and feel the power of these components. Get ready to familiarize yourself with green living because these salves are useful for various common ailments.

It is easy to make salves with your family, but you should keep these salves labeled and sealed in sterile jars. Select cold and dark places to keep them secure. You can use baby food jars to secure them and always use clean utensils to remove slave to avoid transfer of bacteria to your salve with your finger. By keeping your homemade salve clean, you can increase the shelf life of this product.

This book is designed to help you in the preparation of salve. If you want to prepare salves at home, follow the given recipes:

Chapter 1 – Tips to Make Herbal Salves

Salve making is an easy procedure, but you have to focus on some important things to get a clean and herbal product for you and your family.

Carefully Collect Herbs and Essential Oils

For the preparation of salve, you will require several herbs and essential oils. You can use diluted essential oils, but it will be a god to use a combination of infused oils and essential oils. Both types of oils have their benefits.

Herbs to Make Infused Oil

There are a few useful herbs to infuse oils, such as

Plantain Leaves: These leaves are famous to prepare quick healing salves.

Mint Leaves: You should use these leaves to make eczema salve.

Nettle leaves: These leaves are good for anti-allergic salves, and you should wear gloves while handling these leaves. The procedure to use these leaves will be the same as you do with other leaves to make a salve.

Calendula Blossoms: These are perfect for burn and anti-fungal salves. Their salve will be right for the foot of athletes.

Yarrow blossoms: Salve made of these flowers will help you to treat infections and minor bleeding:

Thyme leaves and flowers: You can use them to prepare disinfectant salt for small cuts and scrapes.

Lavender Blossoms: These are useful to disinfect an adolescent skin and reduce oil of this skin.

Leaves of Lemon balm: You can use these leaves for lip gloss and get rid of cold sores due to its anti-viral properties.

Comfrey leaves: You can use these leaves for poorly heal wounds and sprains.

Arnica flowers and leaves: These are good for bruises

Flowering tops of St. John's Wart: If you want to make a disinfectant salve treat burns and cuts, you can use these flowers. Keep it in mind that their salve will work opposite to sunscreen and increase the sensitivity of your skin. If you are using this, keep yourself away from the sun.

Essential Oils for Salve:

You can infuse mint essential oil with mint to make eczema salve. Mint oil has cooling properties and helps you to treat itchy conditions. You can infuse mint oil with nettle, plantain, and calendula as well to use for itchy problems.

Sage, thyme, and pine essential oils can fight with germs and their salves are good for cuts and scrapes.

Lavender oils have a wonderful smell and their mildly disinfectant properties make them suitable to use in an anti-pimple salve for the face.

If you want strong anti-fungal salve, you should use tea tree essential oil. Its smell is not good, but it has numerous benefits for the foot of athletes.

Tips to collect Herbs

To make salve, you should always use fresh herbs free from herbicides and pesticides. Various chemicals of these sprays are highly toxic, and their use is prohibited on medicinal or food crops. If you want to collect fresh herbs from lawns, you should ask the owner about the utilization of this spray. The above-listed herbs are useful for your salves. Selecting an herb locally available in your area will be good. If you find any replacement of these herbs with similar properties, you can use this herb. Before using any plant in your salve, you are responsible for checking their allergic reactions and sensitivity of user's skin.

Most salves require the use of above-ground plants, such as flowers and leaves. It rarely needs pulling up or dig up a plant. You should avoid digging up or pull out and always use clippers or scissors to cut flowers and stems. It will help you to avoid bruising any plant and give it a chance to grow again in 15 days or more.

You should have enough herbs to fill one small jar with its pieces. If you want to use salve for a family, you should use one-quart mason jar of infused oil for each herb. Store herbs in the refrigerator for almost two days before following the next steps or you can dry them for later use. Using fresh herbs in your recipes will be good.

Infused Oil Procedure

In the first step, separate small flowers, such as lavender, yarrow and small leaves like thyme from the stems by holding the stem firmly in your hand. Loosely pull the leaves and flowers and secure them separately. You can cut large blossoms and leaves into ½" pieces.

Put Herbs in Infusing Mason Jars

Your jars should be large enough to hold all herbs easily. If your pot is full of herbs, you can infuse your oils in a better way. Sterilize your mason jars by pouring boiling water or washing them properly through your dishwasher.

Gently pack your jars with chopped herbs and pack them firmly instead of leaving them loose and fluffy. It will make your salve potent.

Pour Oil in Jars

Select base oil for your salve, such as olive oil is good for dry skin, almond oil or lard are also good. You can choose an oil on the basis of the sensitivity of your skin. Pour your preferred base oil in the jars until your selected oil completely covers the herbs. Use a chopstick or butter knife to stab down herbs in a jar and release all air bubbles. You may have to add more oil and keep adding oil until the air bubbles are completely gone, and the mason jars are filled (leave one-inch headspace). The bits of herbs should be under base oil. Cover your jars to avoid any mold growth. Use the back of one spoon to press the stray petals and leaves slowly down toward the surface.

Label Your Jars

Write the name of herb and base oil on a small paper along with the date of filling these jars. Stick this labels on your jars to remember their date and name.

Brew Infused Oil

Slowly close the lid of your mason jars, but don't screw them tight. Keep your pots in a place where direct sunlight falls for a few hours in a day. The sun rays will play an active role to preserve your oil and release the medicinal properties and compounds of herbs in the oil.

Check your oil once on a regular basis and stick chopstick or butter knife to the bottom of each jar to release any bubble and add oil, if needed. Make sure to cover all petals and leaves with oil and securely close the jar again. Wait for almost three weeks and the sun rays will infuse your oil.

Cooking Procedure for Salve

You will complete this step in one day or strain your oil and keep in the refrigerator for almost two weeks before making a salve.

Strain Infused Oil

Take a large piece of cheesecloth (one cheese cloth for one jar of infused oil). Put this material in a bowl and carefully dump the herb-and-oil content of one jar on the cheese cloth. Grasp all the corners of the cheesecloth and lift it in a way to enclose herb material in the cheese cloth. Carefully wrap the top of cheese cloth and squeeze it like a wet cloth to get all oil out of these herbs. You will get a colorful oil, either black, golden, reddish or even light color (depends on the color of herbs).

You can store this strained oil for almost two weeks before making a salve. You should keep this oil in a refrigerator and label it again with date and name.

Heat Your Oil

Take a pan and pour infused oil in this pan. You can make various kinds of salves by heating each oil separately and intensify the properties of every herb. You can make salve by combining different oils to get a salve for general purpose. Keep it in mind that its intensity will be low than a salve prepared with one infused the oil.

Heat oil on low heat and in the meantime, you can prepare other ingredients for salve. Keep an eye on your oil because you shouldn't let it boil. Some herbs may lose their medicinal potency with boiling. Always heat oil on low heat and keep your eye on it.

Caution: Boiling any oil is disreputable with good purpose. It can splatter, catch fire or cause burns.

Add Wax in Salve and Test the Consistency

Once your oil is warm, add some small pieces of bee wax to oil and let them slowly melt. The typical ratio of bee wax is one-ounce wax in one cup oil, but this may vary.

You can start with a few chunk of wax for one quart of herbal oil. Let this wax melt and then remove it from heat. Put one teaspoon of this hot oil on a spoon and keep this spoon in the freezer for almost 3 – 5 minutes to let it cool. Test out the evenness of salve on your hand or other skin. You may require different consistency for various parts of your body. For instance, a lip gloss should be firm enough, and a facial salve can be a bit firm. The salve for scrapes and eczema should be softer, but it should hold a good shape.

If your salve is not thick enough, you can add some pieces of wax and let them melt again. Follow the similar procedure to test this salve again until you are satisfied with the consistency of salve. Turn off heat and remove your pan from stove.

Add Preservatives and Smells

You can add vitamin E and essential oil at this stage because both are heat sensitive. Add them after removing your salve from heat. Add almost 20 – 30 drops of essential oil in half-quart of oil. While adding essential oil, you should keep your face away from the pan because the vapor of hot essential oil can burn your nose and eyes.

Mix one teaspoon of vitamin E or squeeze out 5 to 6 capsules of vitamin E. This vitamin will increase the life of your salve, and diluted vitamin E is good for your skin as well. Be careful and avoid the use of undiluted vitamin E or essential oil on your skin. If you get them accidently on your skin, instantly wash your face to prevent any damage.

Pour Salve in Containers

It is time to pour your hot salve carefully in containers. You shouldn't let it cool in the pan because it will be difficult to remove from the pan. Carefully pour this salve in containers and avoid dropping this hot salve on your skin.

Label and Store Salve Containers

After putting salve in the containers, let it cool down before moving. You should label your salve with name and date immediately. Without a label, you will not be able to identify different salves. Write the date because salves last for six months to one year by storing in dark and cool places. You can use these salves as per your needs, such as treat your burns, infections, cuts, etc.

Chapter 2 – 20 Herbal Salve Recipes for Various Uses

Homemade healing salves are useful to treat cut, stings, bruises, skin irritations and poison. You can use them for the treatment of diaper rashes. There are a few recipes that you can use to make healing salves:

Recipe 01: Standard Salve
- Almond oil or olive oil: 2 cups
- Beeswax pastilles: ¼ cup
- Echinacea root: 1 teaspoon
- Comfrey leaf (dry): 2 tablespoons
- Plantain leaf (dry): 2 tablespoons
- Yarrow flower: 1 teaspoon
- Calendula flowers (dry): 1 tablespoon
- Rosemary leaf (dry): 1 teaspoon

Directions:

In the first step, infuse herbs in oil by combining herbs in an airtight jar and leave for almost 3 to 4 weeks in a place with plenty of sunlight. Shake on a regular basis. If you don't want to infuse with this procedure, you can heat herbs in olive oil on low heat in one double boiler for almost 3 hours. The oil should turn green.

Strain herbs out of this oil through cheesecloth and carefully squeeze oil of all herbs. Discard herbs and heat infused oil in your double boiler with small parts of beeswax. Let the beeswax melt and mix them well. Test the consistency of oil as stated in the previous chapter and pour into small jars and tubes. You can use this salve on cuts, stings, poison ivy, bites, wounds and diaper rashes.

Recipe 02: All-purpose Healing Salve
- Coconut oil: 1 cup
- Olive oil: 1 cup
- Beeswax Pastilles: 4 tablespoons
- Vitamin E oil: ½ teaspoon
- 4 oz mason jars

For Each Jar
- Lavender oil: 10 drops
- Lemon oil: 8 drops
- Melaleuca: 6 drops
- Vitamin E oil: ½ teaspoon

Directions:

Take a pot and melt olive oil, beeswax and coconut oil in a warm bath (pour these ingredients into a glass jar and put in a pot half filled with water). Stir with one knife frequently until melted. It will take almost 15 minutes because you have to melt on low heat.

Mix all essential oils & vitamin E and pour in one glass jar (the quantity given above is for one jar only). Put a cheesecloth or paper towel on the jar with essential oil and strain melted mixture, and let them cool. Cover with lid and keep in a secure place. The shelf life of this salve is eight months because vitamin oil is added. It will be good to put this mixture in small jars to easily carry these jars with you while traveling.

Recipe 03: Basic Recipe for Salve

The basic salve will carry your herbs that you will add in the oil. There is are some simple way to make your basic salve:

1. Prepare a mixture of five parts oil and 1-part beeswax
2. Combine 2-part beeswax with four parts lanolin or lard and 1-part oil.
3. Combine four parts shea butter, cocoa butter and combine with one-part oil and beeswax (one part).

Procedure to Make Salve:

Melt your ingredients on low heat and stir as they blend well. Add herbal infusion or herbs of your choice. Pour this mixture into a container and let it cool.

Herbal Infused Oil

- Dried herbs: 1 part
- Oil: 2 parts

Directions:

Mix herbs and oil in a container and release all bubbles in the oil. Pack your container with herbs and oil tightly and put in a warm place for almost three weeks to infuse the oil. Shake this oil with a chopstick on a regular basis and once the herbs are completely infused, strain them in a glass container through a cheese cloth. Store in a dark and cool place in an airtight jar before making a salve. It should be used within two weeks.

Recipe 04: First Aid Salve

- Gold essential oil: 1 part
- Calendula oil: 1 part
- Comfrey Oil: 1 part
- Lavender Oil: 1 drop
- Tea tree oil: 1/8 teaspoon
- Vitamin E: 800IU

Directions:

In the first step, infuse herbs in oil by combining herbs in an airtight jar and leave for almost 3 to 4 weeks in a place with plenty of sunlight. Shake on a regular basis. If you don't want to infuse with this procedure, you can heat herbs in olive oil on low heat in one double boiler for almost 3 hours. The oil should turn green. Strain herbs out of this oil through cheesecloth and carefully squeeze oil of all herbs. Discard herbs and heat infused oil in your double boiler with small parts of beeswax. Let the beeswax melt and mix them well. Test the consistency of oil as stated in the previous chapter and pour into small jars and tubes. You can use this salve on cuts, stings, poison ivy, bites, wounds and diaper rashes.

Recipe 05: Diaper Rash Salve

- Lavender Oil: 1 part
- Calendula Oil: 1 part

- Comfrey Oil: 1 part
- Vitamin E: 800 IU
- Combine 2-part beeswax with four parts lanolin or lard and 1-part oil.

Directions:

Follow standard or basic recipe to prepare diaper rash salve.

Note: To get equal parts, you can use a measuring cup instead of weighing these ingredients.

Recipe 06: Burn Salve
- Calendula Flowers: 1 part
- Comfrey Leaves: 1 part
- Comfrey Root: 1 part
- Saint-John's Wort-Flowers: 1 part
- Olive Oil: 1 part
- Grated Beeswax

Directions:

Put comfrey leaves, wort flowers and Calendula flowers in the upper section of boiler along with your olive oil. Fill the bottom of the boiler with water and let it boil on low heat. Let them gently simmer for almost 30 to 60 minutes. Check them frequently to ensure that oil is not overheating. If you notice smoke, it means the oil is overheating.

Strain this oil and put in a small pan. Add ¼ cup of grated beeswax in 1 cup infused the oil. Heat these ingredients on low flame until the beeswax is completely melted. Turn off heat and test the small amount of consistency by putting in your freezer. If it looks hard and difficult to spread, add more oil and heat it again. If it is oily, add extra beeswax and heat it again. Once you get desired consistency, you can pour this mixture into glass jars and store properly in cool and dark places for several months.

Recipe 07: Cuticle Balm
- Coconut oil: 1 tablespoon
- Almond oil: 1 tablespoon
- Hemp oil: 1 tablespoon
- Mango butter: 1 tablespoon
- Grated beeswax: 1 ½ tablespoon

Essential Oils:
- Lavender EO: 10 drops
- Peppermint EO: 5 drops
- Eucalyptus EO: 5 drops
- Fennel EO: 5 drops
- Clary sage EO: 5 drops

Directions:

You should arrange double boiler, a metal spoon, and metal pots or tins. Melt mango butter, beeswax and oils in a double boiler. Remove from heat and add essential oils. Mix them well and pour them into pots and let them cooled down.

Recipe 08: Herbal Infused Balm
- Dry Herbs (chamomile + peppermint + Calendula and Lavender)
- Carrier Oil (Jojoba, Almond or Olive)
- Beeswax: 2 tablespoons for ¼ cup oil
- Essential oils of your choice
- Lidded containers

Directions:

Infuse oils for almost 2 to 3 weeks in airtight containers. You should toss them on a regular basis. Strain out herbs and combine this oil in a saucepan with beeswax and add in a double broiler to melt on low heat. Once melted, pour these ingredients into clean containers and mix 20 to 30 drops of essential oils in each container. Let this salve cool down and turn hard. Store in cool and dry places.

Recipe 09: Foot Salve
- Pure lanolin: 4 oz.
- Raw beeswax: 1 oz.
- Olive oil (infuse this oil with calendula flowers, comfrey leaves, and plantain leaves): 1.5 oz.
- Shea butter: .5 oz.
- Cocoa butter: .25 oz.
- Neem oil: 1/2 teaspoon
- Sea buckthorn oil: 1/4 teaspoon
- Vitamin-E oil: 1ml

- Lavender EO (essential oil): 1ml
- Rosemary EO: 1ml
- Fir needle EO: 1ml
- Tea tree EO: 1ml
- Rosemary extract: 1ml

Directions:

To prepare this salve, you have to follow the standard procedure given in the first chapter to make a salve. Carefully follow each and every step. You can use a boiler to melt beeswax and oil, but you should keep it on low heat.

Recipe 10: Charcoal Black Salve
- Calendula-infused oil: 1/4 cup (prepare your infused oil)
- Coconut oil: 1/4 cup
- Beeswax (beeswax pellets): 2 teaspoons
- Activated charcoal (almost 15 capsules): 3 teaspoons
- Clay (bentonite clay): 3 teaspoons
- Lavender EO: 10 drops
- Tea tree EO: 10 drops

Directions:

Melt coconut oil and beeswax together by putting your glass container in a saucepan filled with water. Place this saucepan on low flame and let it melt. Make sure to use only glass container because the plastic container is not good for this purpose. After melting, turn off heat and add remaining ingredients. Let the salve cool down until it becomes hard. Secure them in lidded containers in dark and cool places.

You can apply this salve directly on splinter area, bug bite and sting. Apply salve on your skin after every 12 hours until needed.

Recipe 11: Perfect Salve for Burn

- Raw Honey: ¼ cup
- Coconut oil (extra virgin): 1 tablespoon
- Aloe vera: 1 tablespoon

Directions:

Whisk these ingredients together with a mixer or a spoon. Store this salve in a glass jar. Before using this salve, clean the affected area with apple vinegar. It will help you to restore the minerals and vitamin of your skin. Apply this burn salve on cleansed area and cover with a gauze to keep this salve on your skin. This salve is for minor burns, so avoid its use on major wounds that require immediate medical attention.

Recipe 12: Plantain Salve

- Olive oil (infused with dry plantain): 4 ounces
- Beeswax: 1 ounce
- Grapefruit seed (Extract): 5 drops
- Vitamin-E oil: 5 drops
- Chopstick containers, tins or glass jars to hold slave

- Peppermint Oil: 2 drops
- Lavender Oil: 2 drops

Directions:

Follow the standard procedure given in the first chapter to infuse the oil and make your salve. Carefully pour prepared salve in glass containers and let them set for almost 24 hours. Make sure to select an airtight jar to keep them secure for a longer period.

Recipe 13: Dandelion Salve
- Dandelion infused-oil: 3.5 ounces
- Beeswax Pastilles: 0.5 ounces

Directions:

You have to follow a standard procedure of making a salve and add a few drops of essential oils and Vitamin-E oil in salve at the end. This salve is useful for arthritis and achy joints, chapped and rough skin and sore muscles.

Recipe 14: Sore Muscles Salve
- Heat-safe bowl
- Small saucepan
- Coconut oil: 1/4 cup
- Olive oil: 1/4 cup
- Beeswax: 1 tablespoon
- Ground pepper: 1/4 teaspoon

- Ground ginger: 1/4 teaspoon
- Peppermint EO: 20 drops
- Eucalyptus EO: 20 drops
- Clove oil: 20 drops
- Strainer
- Coffee filter
- Sealable container
- Small bowl

Directions:

Fill your saucepan with water and put a heatproof bowl inside this saucepan. In the absence of heatproof bowl, you can use a clean can as well. Add olive oil and coconut oil in this bowl and sprinkle ginger and ground pepper in the oil. Let the water simmer to keep this mixture warm for almost 20 minutes in hot water.

After 20 minutes, add oils and beeswax. Let them completely melt. Put one strainer in a small bowl and add a coffee filter on this strainer. Carefully pour oil and butter mixture over this strainer. It will help you to get a clean salve. Add eucalyptus and peppermint essential oils to this mixture and mix them with a chopstick. Carefully pour this warming salve in small containers and leave them at room temperature for various hours. Seal these bottles and store in cool and dry places. You can use them on your sore muscles as per your need. You shouldn't use it on your face and properly wash your hands after its use to avoid interaction with nose, mouth, and eyes.

Recipe 15: Pepper Salve for Joint and Arthritis
- Cayenne powder: 3 tablespoons

- Grapeseed oil: 1 cup (you can also use jojoba oil, almond oil or olive oil)

- Grated beeswax: ½ cup

- Double boiler

- Sealable glass jars

Directions:

Mix three tablespoons cayenne powder with one cup oil and heat in your double boiler for almost 5 to 10 minutes on medium heat. Mix ½ cup grated beeswax and stir well to melt it completely. Make sure to mix all ingredients together. Put this mixture in your refrigerator for almost ten minutes and whisk them together. Chill for 10 to 15 minutes and whip again before putting this mixture in a glass jar. Secure its lid on its place and store in the refrigerator. You can secure it for 1 ½ week and use to relieve pain. You shouldn't use it on your face.

Recipe 16: Chest Rub
- Rosemary oil: 1 part

- Thyme oil: 1 part

- Infused Peppermint oil: 1 part

- Camphor EO: ½ teaspoon

- Eucalyptus EO: ½ teaspoon

Directions:

You can use any standard recipe to make this salve and add beeswax as per your needs.

Recipe 17: Hemorrhoid Salve
- Calendula oil: 1 part
- Comfrey oil: 1 part
- Nettle leaf (oil): 1 part
- Marshmallow root (oil): ½ part
- Powdered myrrh: 2 teaspoons
- Lavender oil: 1 part
- Vitamin E: 800 IU

Directions:

You can use any standard recipe to make this salve and add beeswax as per your needs.

Recipe 18: Salve for Gardener
- Comfrey oil: 3 parts
- Calendula oil: 3 parts
- St John's wort-oil: 3 parts
- Plantain oil: 2 parts
- Vitamin-E oil: 1 part

Directions:

You can use any base oil to make a salve and follow the standard recipe to make this salve. You can rub this salve on psoriasis, calluses, and dry skin.

Recipe 19: Lip Salve
- Lavender Oil: 1 part
- Comfrey Oil: 1 part
- Rose Oil: 1 part
- Vitamin-E oil: 800IU

Directions:

Follow standard recipes and use coconut oil and Combine 2-part beeswax with four parts lanolin or lard and 1-part oil. Coconut oil is good for your lips. You can keep this salve slightly soft to apply easily on your lips.

Recipe 20: Super-Strength Salve for Pain
- Beeswax: 1 cup
- Habanero powder: 4 tablespoons
- Grapeseed oil, olive oil or jojoba oil: 4 cups
- Gloves
- Double boiler
- Glass jar with secure lid

Directions:

Combine habanero powder and grapeseed oil or other oil of your choice in one double boiler. Let this mixture warm for almost 5 to 10 minutes on medium heat.

Add 1 cup beeswax to this mixture and stir them constantly to melt beeswax and mix with other ingredients. Let it chill for almost ten minutes in your refrigerator and whisk them together. Chill for another ten minutes and whisk again before pouring into a glass container. Seal its lid and keep in a refrigerator. You can use it for 1 ½ weeks. Apply on particular areas to treat pain. You shouldn't use it on your face.

Conclusion

These healing salves are healthy for everyone to use. You can keep your hand moisture with the use of salve and heal irritated and chap skin, lips, and heels. These rubs are good to soothe sunburn, welts, and burns. These are based on natural ingredients that are easily available in the grocery stores. You should be careful while shopping these ingredients because some of these ingredients can be harmful to your skin. If you have allergy with any particular ingredient, you can replace it with a safe alternative.

You will use essential oils and Vitamin-E oil in each recipe; therefore, you can keep them secure for 8 to 12 months. There will be no burden on your budget, and it is safe for your whole family. You can prepare rubs and send them as a gift to your friends and family members. It will be a cheap and healthy gift for your family members. You can fill small containers and tubes with a salve to carry them easily in your handbag along you. The use of essential oils and healthy ingredients will help you to enhance your beauty and protect your skin.

Made in United States
Troutdale, OR
01/02/2024